HUMAN BODY PARTS
ANATOMY
COLORING BOOK

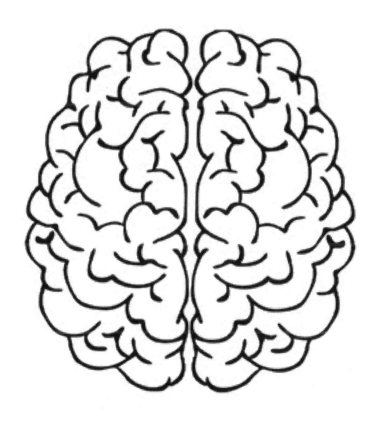

BELONGS TO

_____

_____

This book offers diverse illustrations of the human (male and female) body anatomy, lots of black and white drawings to color, As well as the names of deferent organs of the body. The book also includs pages with definitions for each organ.

The cell

is the basic structural, functional, and biological unit of all known organisms. A cell is the smallest unit of life. Cells are often called the "building blocks of life". The study of cells is called cell biology, cellular biology, or cytology.

Cell

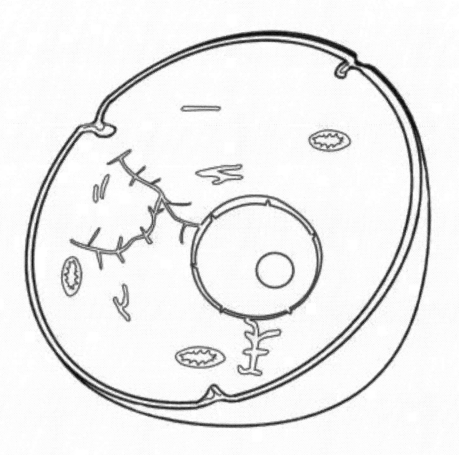

Eukaryote

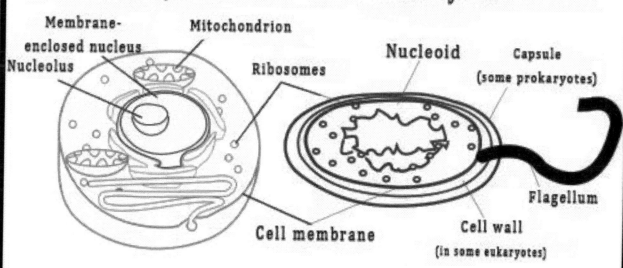

Membrane-enclosed nucleus

Mitochondrion

Nucleolus

Ribosomes

Cell membrane

Prokaryote

Nucleoid

Capsule
(some prokaryotes)

Flagellum

Cell wall
(in some eukaryotes)

The Head

Is the upper portion of the body, consisting of the skull with its coverings and contents, including the lower jaw. It is attached to the spinal column by way of the first cervical vertebra, the atlas, and connected with the trunk of the body by the muscles, blood vessels, and nerves that constitute the neck.

Head

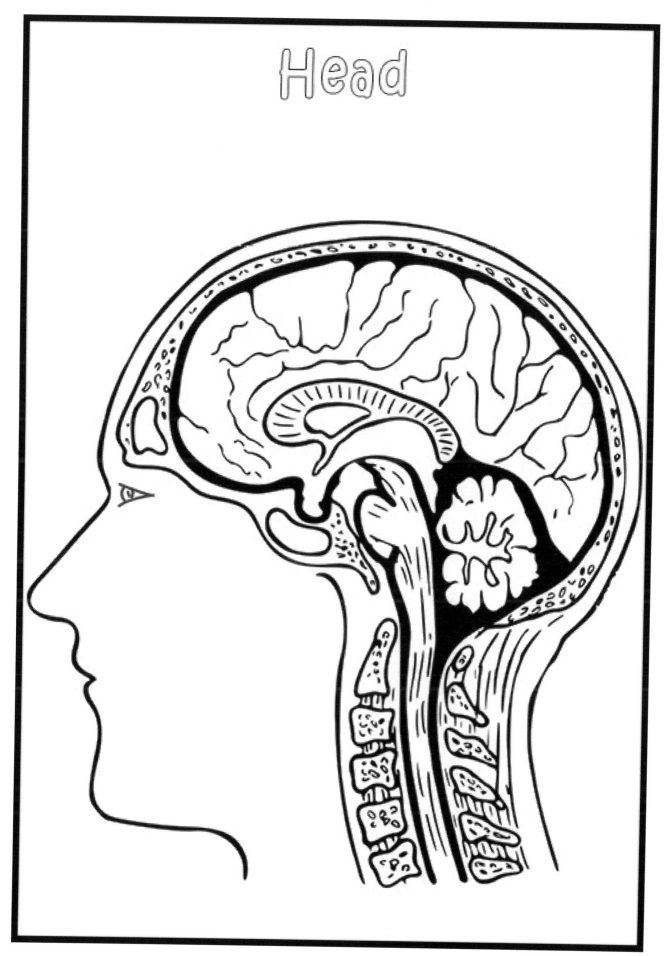

The skull

The skull is a bony structure that forms the head in vertebrates. It supports the structures of the face and provides a protective cavity for the brain. The skull is composed of two parts: the cranium and the mandible. In humans, these two parts are the neurocranium and the viscerocranium or facial skeleton.

Skull

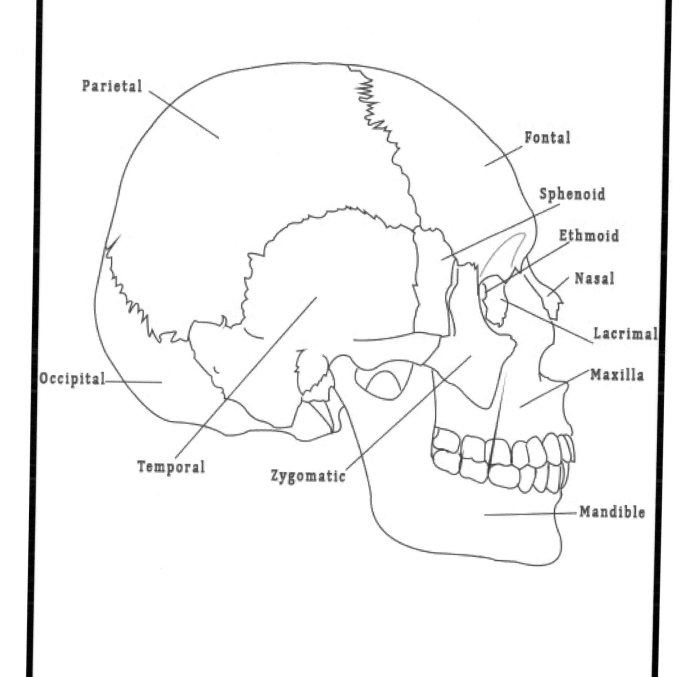

Parietal

Fontal

Sphenoid

Ethmoid

Nasal

Lacrimal

Maxilla

Occipital

Temporal

Zygomatic

Mandible

The **brain**

is the organ that serves as the center of the nervous system. It is located in the head, usually close to the sensory organs for senses such as vision. It is the most complex organ in a the human body.

Brain structure

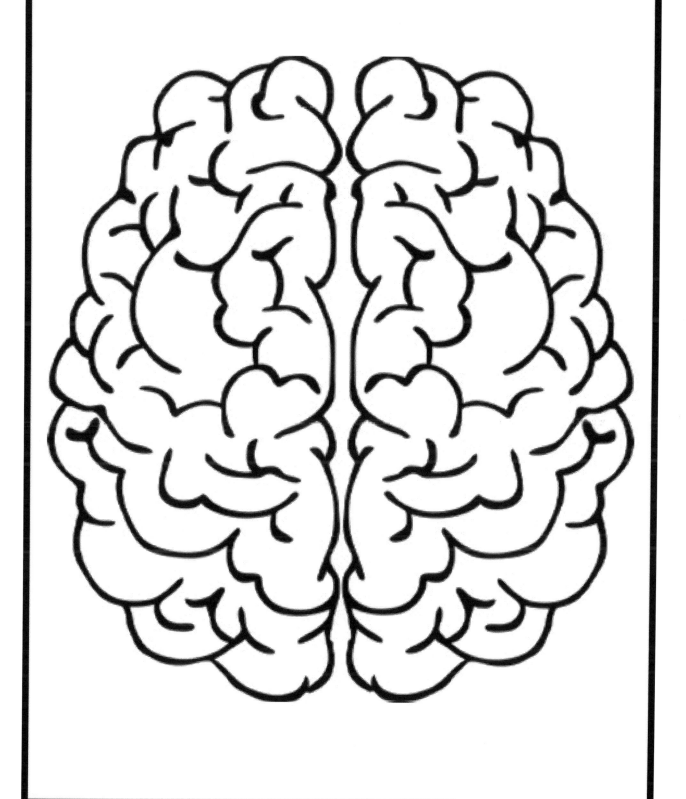

The **eye**

is an organ of the visual system. They provide Humans with vision, the ability to receive and process visual detail, as well as enabling several photo response functions that are independent of vision.

Eye

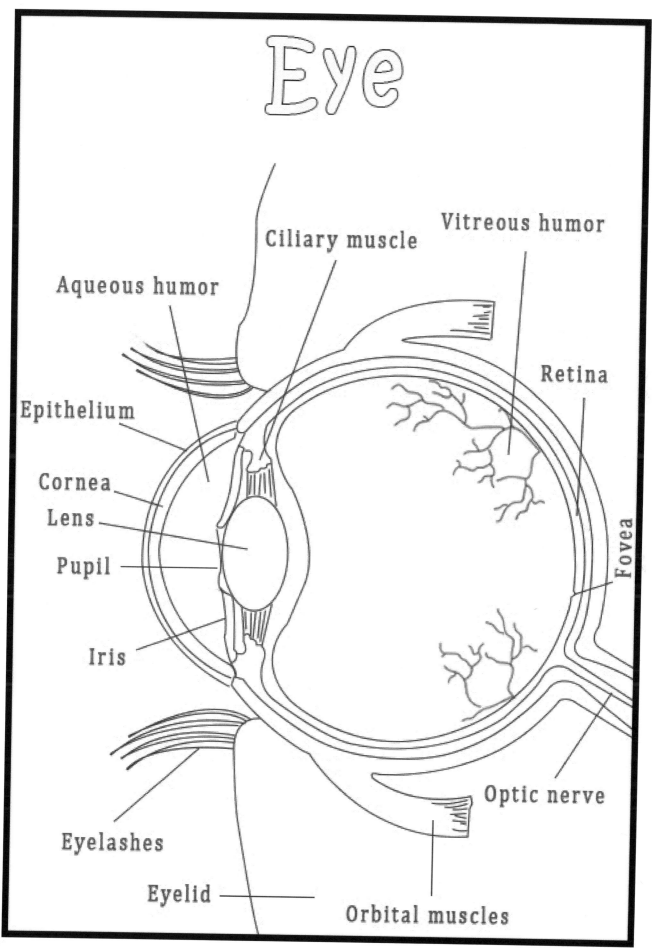

Ciliary muscle

Vitreous humor

Aqueous humor

Retina

Epithelium

Cornea

Lens

Pupil

Fovea

Iris

Optic nerve

Eyelashes

Eyelid

Orbital muscles

10

The **ear**

Is the organ of hearing.
It develops from the
first pharyngeal pouch
and six small swellings
that develop in the early
embryo called otic
placodes, which are
derived from ectoderm..

Ear

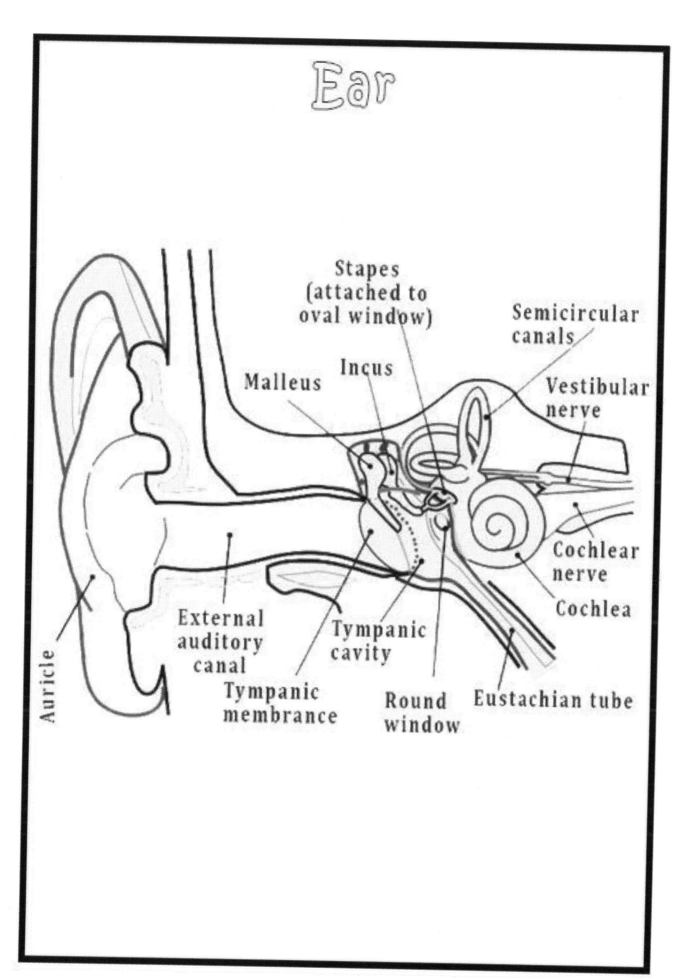

The mouth

is the first portion of the alimentary canal that receives food and produces saliva. The oral mucosa is the mucous membrane epithelium lining the inside of the mouth.

Mouth
(Anterior view)

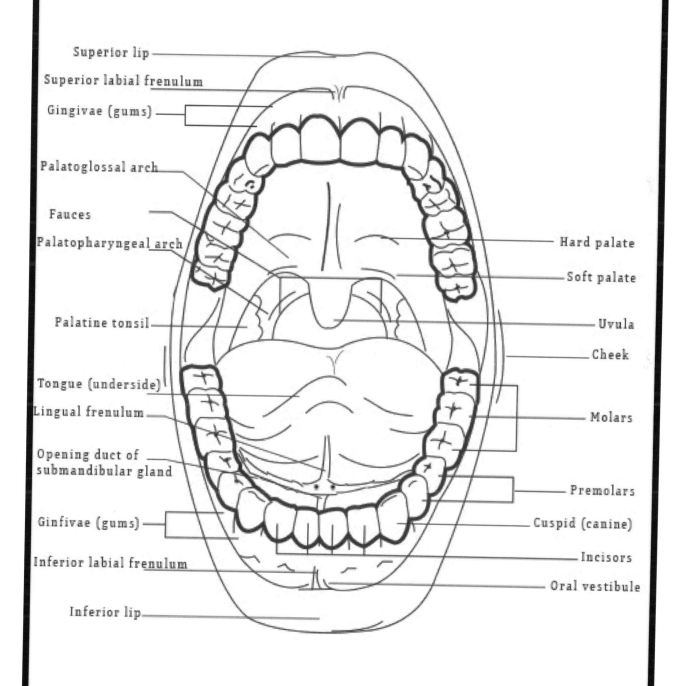

Superior lip

Superior labial frenulum

Gingivae (gums)

Palatoglossal arch

Fauces

Palatopharyngeal arch

Palatine tonsil

Tongue (underside)

Lingual frenulum

Opening duct of
submandibular gland

Ginfivae (gums)

Inferior labial frenulum

Inferior lip

Hard palate

Soft palate

Uvula

Cheek

Molars

Premolars

Cuspid (canine)

Incisors

Oral vestibule

The **tooth**

function to mechanically break down items of food by cutting and crushing them in preparation for swallowing and digesting. Humans have four types of teeth: incisors, canines, premolars, and molars.

Tooth

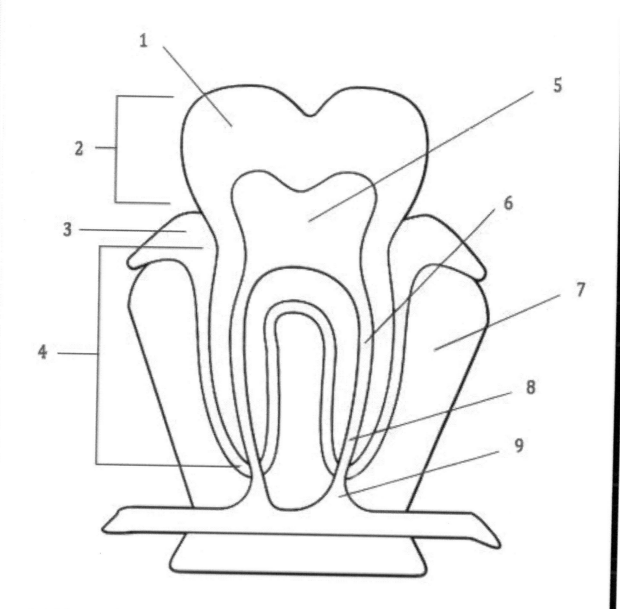

1- Enamel

2- Crown

3- Gum

4 - Root

5- Pulp

6- Root Canal

7- Bone

8- Nerves

9- Blood Vessels

The **tongue**

is a muscular organ in the mouth of most vertebrates that manipulates food for mastication and is used in the act of swallowing. It has importance in the digestive system and is the primary organ of taste in the gustatory system.

Tongue

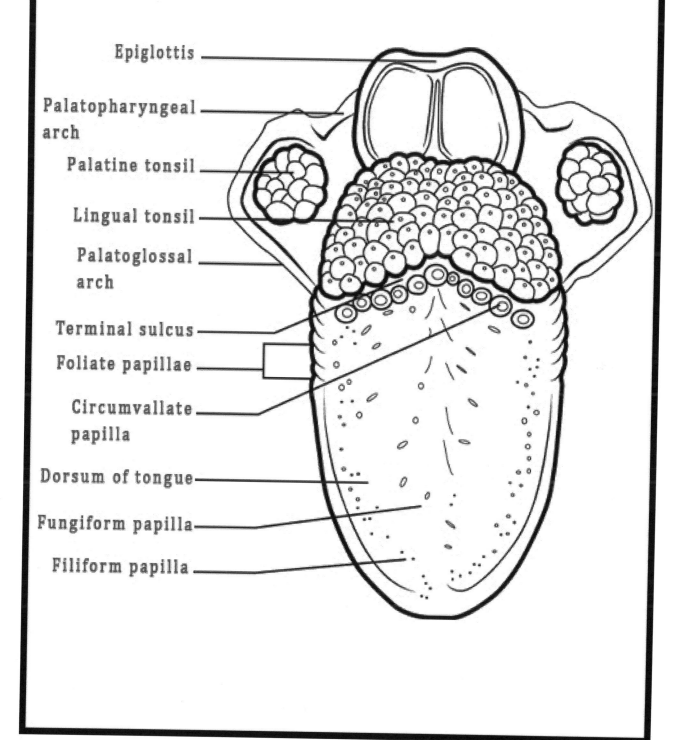

Epiglottis

Palatopharyngeal arch

Palatine tonsil

Lingual tonsil

Palatoglossal arch

Terminal sulcus

Foliate papillae

Circumvallate papilla

Dorsum of tongue

Fungiform papilla

Filiform papilla

The **hair**

is a protein filament
that grows from follicles
found in the dermis.
Hair is one of the
defining characteristics
of mammals. The human
body, apart from areas
of glabrous skin, is
covered in follicles
which produce thick
terminal and fine vellus
hair.

Hair

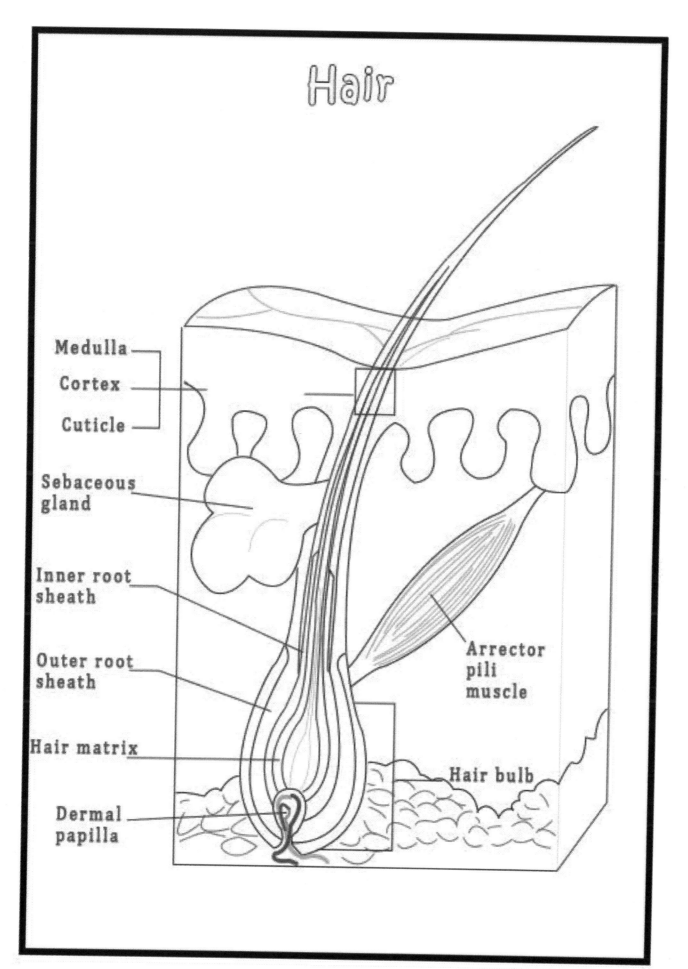

Medulla
Cortex
Cuticle

Sebaceous
gland

Inner root
sheath

Outer root
sheath

Hair matrix

Dermal
papilla

Arrector
pili
muscle

Hair bulb

The neck

is the part of the body on many vertebrates that connects the head with the torso and provides the mobility and movements of the head. The structures of the human neck are anatomically grouped into four compartments: vertebral, visceral and two vascular compartments.

Neck

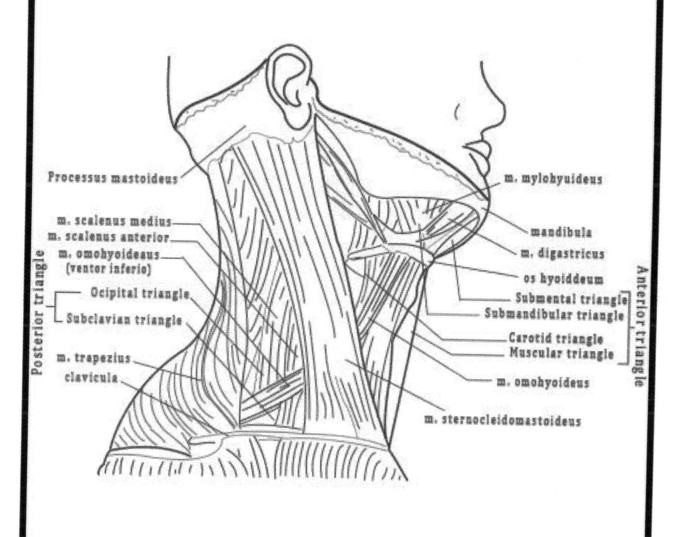

Processus mastoideus

m. scalenus medius
m. scalenus anterior
m. omohyoideaus
(ventor inferio)

Posterior triangle
Ocipital triangle
Subclavian triangle

m. trapezius
clavicula

m. mylohyuideus

mandibula
m. digastricus
os hyoiddeum

Submental triangle
Submandibular triangle

Anterior triangle
Carotid triangle
Muscular triangle

m. omohyoideus

m. sternocleidomastoideus

The **body**

The body is the structure of a human being. It is composed of many different types of cells that together create tissues and subsequently organ systems. They ensure homeostasis and the viability of the human body.

It comprises a head, neck, trunk (which includes the thorax and abdomen), arms and hands, legs and feet.

Man body

(Anterior view) (Posterior view)

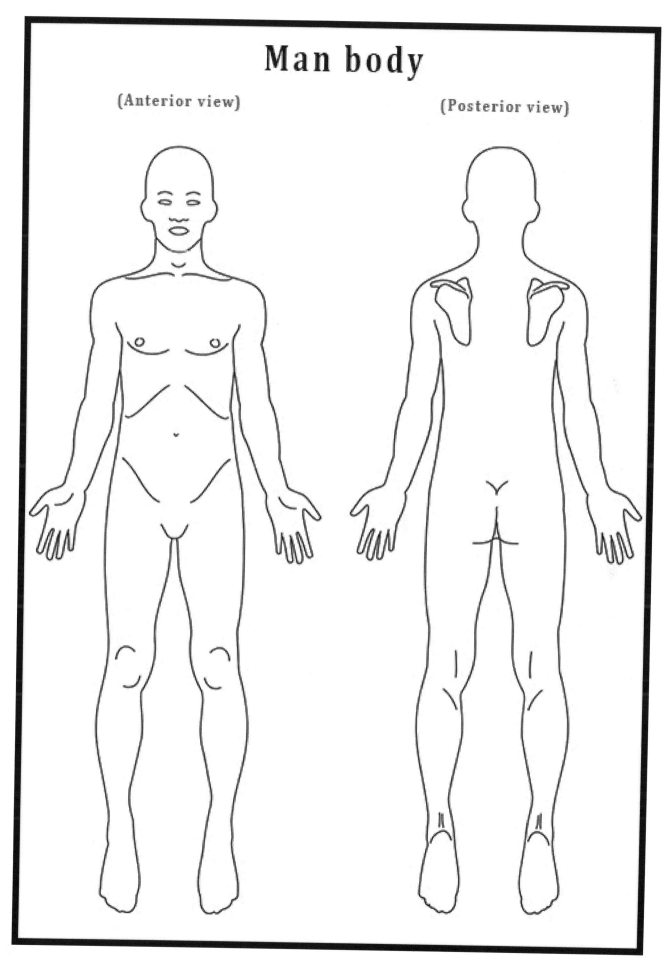

The **body**

is composed of elements
including hydrogen,
oxygen, carbon, calcium
and phosphorus. These
elements reside in
trillions of cells and non-
cellular components of
the body.

Body muscles
(Anterior view)

The body

varies anatomically in known ways. Physiology focuses on the systems and organs of the human body and their functions. Many systems and mechanisms interact in order to maintain homeostasis, with safe levels of substances such as sugar and oxygen in the blood.

Body muscles
(Posterior view)

The **body cavity**

is any space or compartment, or potential space in the body. Cavities accommodate organs and other structures; cavities as potential spaces contain fluid.

The two largest human body cavities are the ventral body cavity, and the dorsal body cavity. In the dorsal body cavity the brain and spinal cord are located.

Cavities of the body

Cranial cavity

Thoracic cavity

Dorsal cavity

Spinal cavity

Ventral cavity

Abdominal cavity

Pelvic cavity

Abdominopelvic cavity

The **rib cage**

Or thoracic cage, is a bony and cartilaginous structure which surrounds the thoracic cavity and supports the shoulder girdle to form the core part of the human skeleton.

Ribs

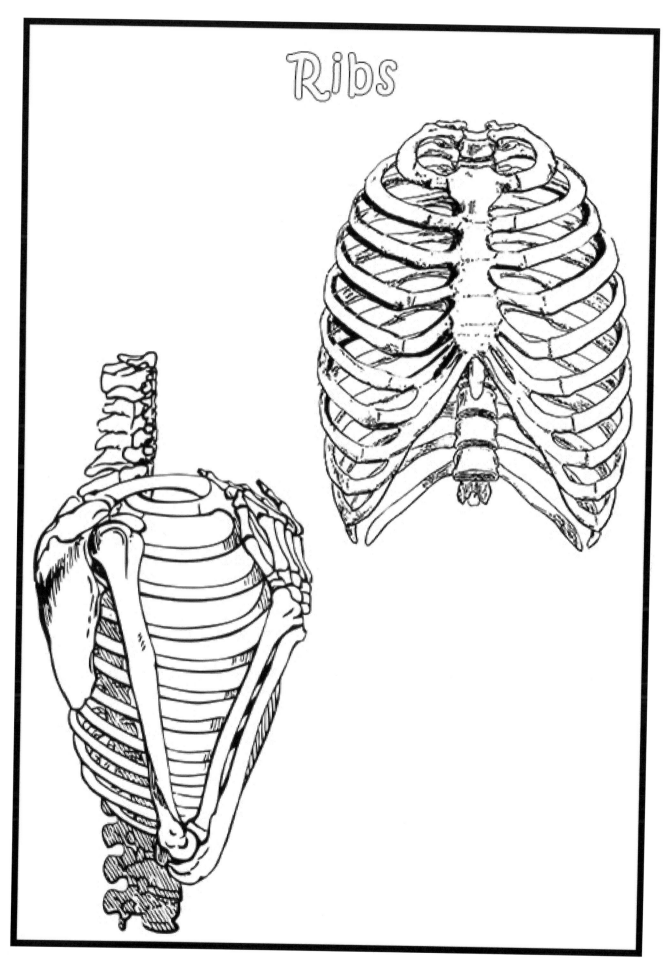

The **organs**

structured collections of cells with a specific function, mostly sit within the body, with the exception of skin. Many organs reside within cavities within the body.

Human Organs

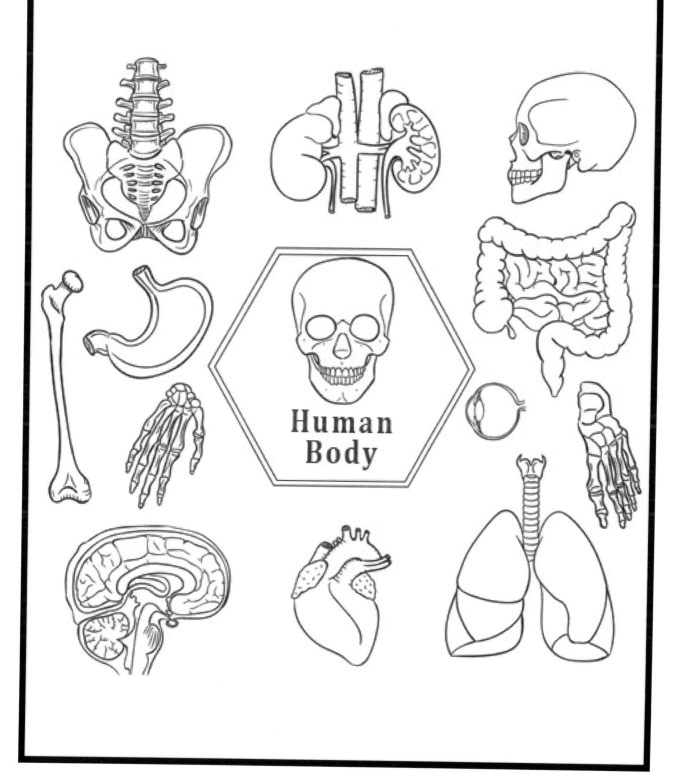

Human
Body

The basic organs

include the heart,

lungs,

liver,

stomach.

Basic Organs of the body

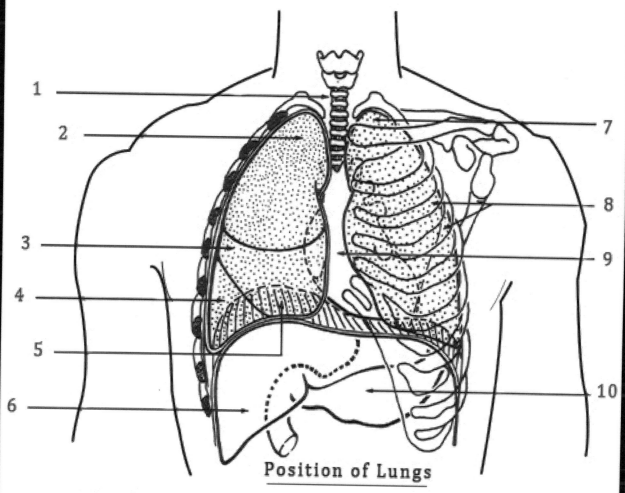

Position of Lungs

1- Trachea

2- Upper lobe (Right lung)

3- Middle lobe

4- Lower lobe

5- Dome of Diaphragm

6- Liver

7- Apex (Left lung)

8- Ribs

9- Heart

10- Stomach

The **heart**

is a muscular organ, which pumps blood through the blood vessels of the circulatory system. Blood provides the body with oxygen and nutrients, as well as assisting in the removal of metabolic wastes. the heart is located between the lungs, in the middle compartment of the chest.

Heart

Aorta

Superior
Vena Cava

Pulmonary
Artery

Right
Artrium

Left
Arteium

Right
Ventricle

Pilmonary
Veins

Inferior
Vena Cava

Left
Ventricle

The **heart**

is divided into four chambers: upper left and right atria and lower left and right ventricles. Commonly the right atrium and ventricle are referred together as the *right heart* and their left counterparts as the *left heart.*

How Does The Heart Work?

To Upper Body

Aorta

Superior Vena Cava

Pulmonary Artery

To Right Lung

To Left Lung

From Left Lung

From Right Lung

Right Atrium

Left Atrium

Right Ventricle

Left Ventricle

Inferior Vena Cava

From Lower Body

To Lower Body

The respiratory system

is a biological system consisting of specific organs and structures used for gas exchange.
the anatomy of a typical respiratory system is the respiratory tract. The tract is divided into an upper and a lower respiratory tract. The upper tract includes the nose, nasal cavities, sinuses, pharynx and the part of the larynx above the vocal folds. The lower tract includes the lower part of the larynx, the trachea, bronchi, bronchioles and the alveoli.

Respiratory system

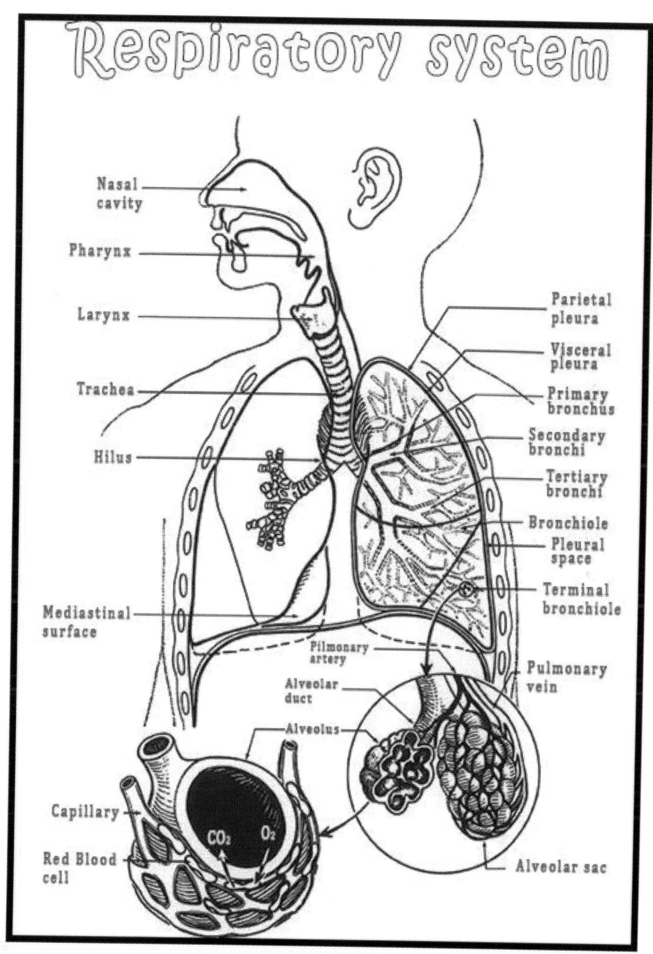

Nasal cavity

Pharynx

Larynx

Trachea

Hilus

Mediastinal surface

Parietal pleura

Visceral pleura

Primary bronchus

Secondary bronchi

Tertiary bronchi

Bronchiole

Pleural space

Terminal bronchiole

Pulmonary artery

Pulmonary vein

Alveolar duct

Alveolus

Capillary

CO_2 O_2

Red Blood cell

Alveolar sac

The liver

is an organ only found in vertebrates which detoxifies various metabolites, synthesizes proteins and produces biochemicals necessary for digestion and growth. it is located in the right upper quadrant of the abdomen, below the diaphragm. Its other roles in metabolism include the regulation of glycogen storage, decomposition of red blood cells and the production of hormones.

The pancreas

is an organ of the digestive system and endocrine system of vertebrates. In humans, it is located in the abdomen behind the stomach and functions as a gland. The pancreas has both an endocrine and a digestive exocrine function.

Liver and Pancreas

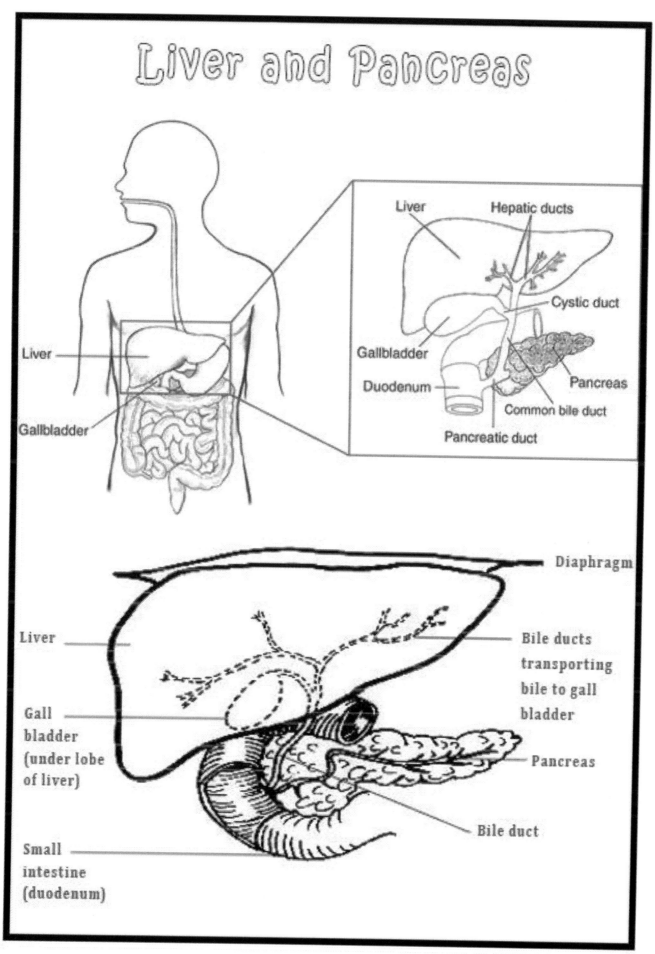

Liver

Gallbladder

Liver

Hepatic ducts

Cystic duct

Gallbladder

Duodenum

Pancreas

Common bile duct

Pancreatic duct

Diaphragm

Liver

Bile ducts transporting bile to gall bladder

Gall bladder (under lobe of liver)

Pancreas

Bile duct

Small intestine (duodenum)

The kidneys

are two bean-shaped organs found in humans. They are located on the left and right in the retroperitoneal space, and in adult humans are about 11 centimeters (4.3 in) in length. They receive blood from the paired renal arteries; blood exits into the paired renal veins. Each kidney is attached to a ureter, a tube that carries excreted urine to the bladder.

Kidney

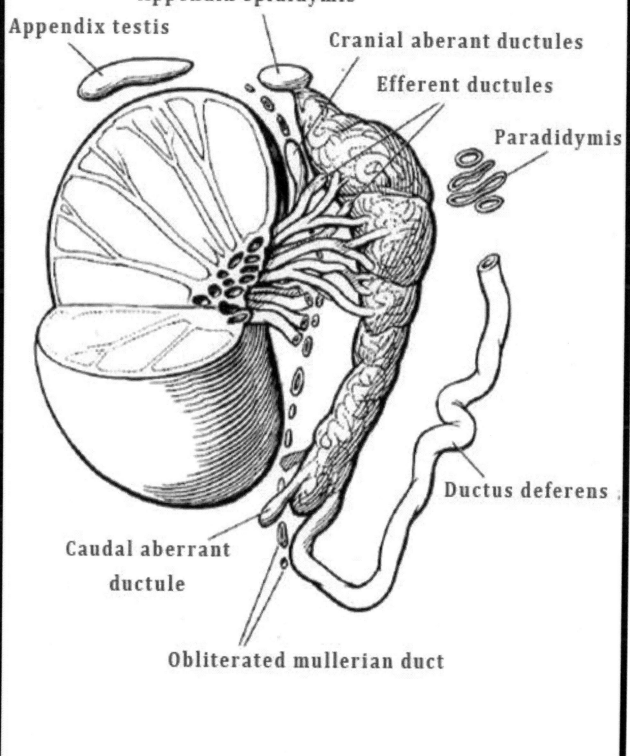

Appendix testis

Appendix epididymis

Cranial aberant ductules

Efferent ductules

Paradidymis

Ductus deferens

Caudal aberrant ductule

Obliterated mullerian duct

The human digestive system

consists of the gastrointestinal tract plus the accessory organs of digestion (the tongue, salivary glands, pancreas, liver, and gallbladder). Digestion involves the breakdown of food into smaller and smaller components, until they can be absorbed and assimilated into the body

Digestive System

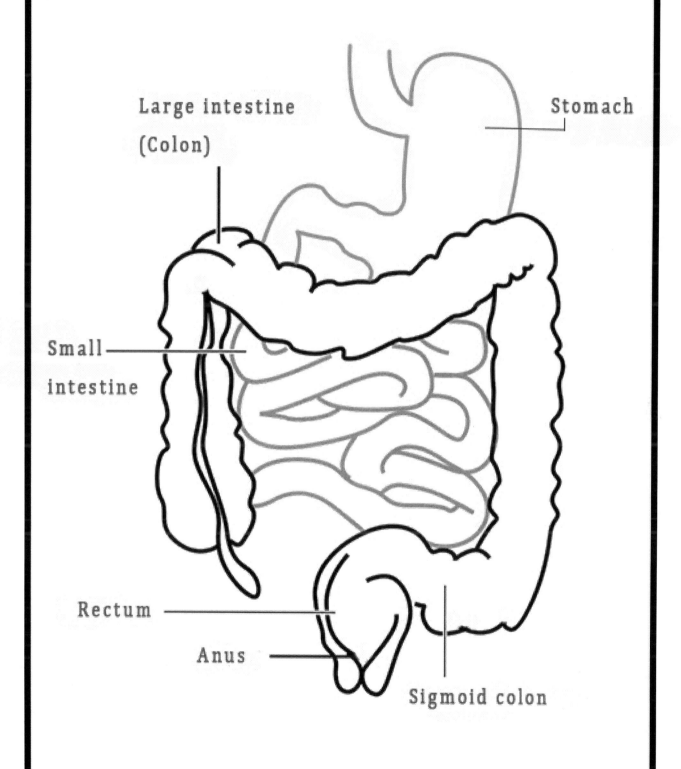

Large intestine
(Colon)

Stomach

Small
intestine

Rectum

Anus

Sigmoid colon

The digestive system

The largest structure of the digestive system is the gastrointestinal tract (GI tract). This starts at the mouth and ends at the anus, covering a distance of about nine (9) meters. The largest part of the GI tract is the colon or large intestine. Water is absorbed here and the remaining waste matter is stored prior to defecation.

Digestive system

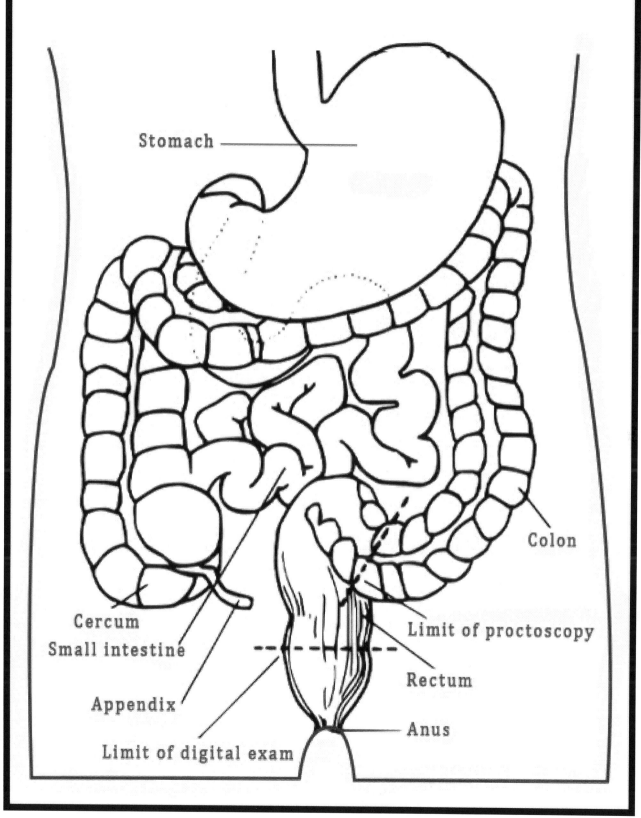

Stomach

Colon

Cercum

Small intestine

Limit of proctoscopy

Appendix

Rectum

Limit of digital exam

Anus

The **digestive system**

There are several organs and other components involved in the digestion of food. The organs known as the accessory digestive organs are the liver, gall bladder and pancreas. Other components include the mouth, salivary glands, tongue, teeth and epiglottis.

Digestive System Parts

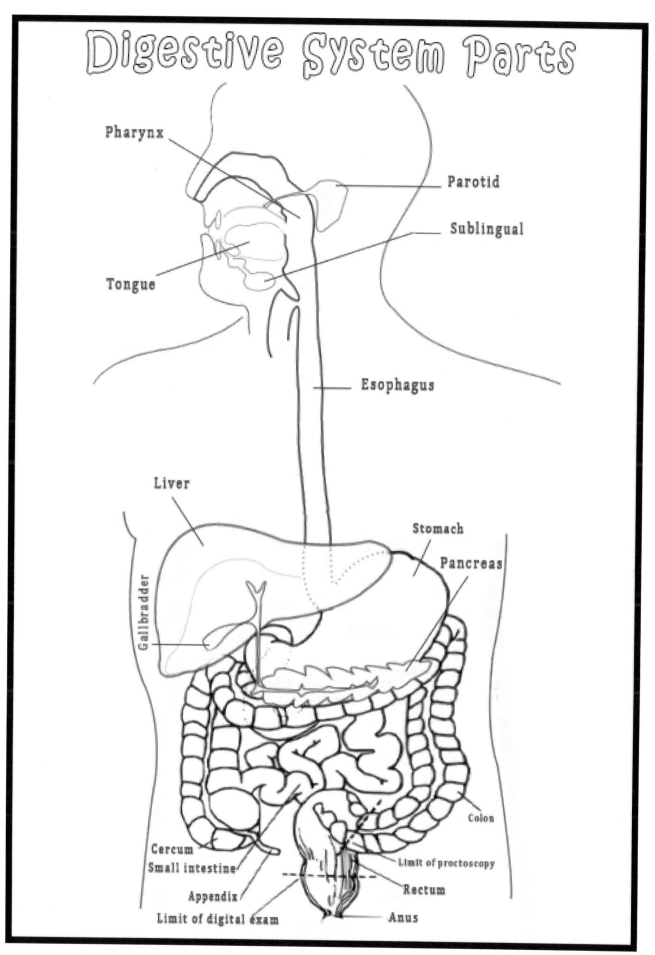

Pharynx

Parotid

Sublingual

Tongue

Esophagus

Liver

Stomach

Pancreas

Gallbladder

Cercum

Small intestine

Appendix

Limit of digital exam

Colon

Limit of proctoscopy

Rectum

Anus

The stomach

is a muscular, hollow organ in the gastrointestinal tract of humans. The stomach has a dilated structure and functions as a vital digestive organ. In the digestive system the stomach is a major organ, it is involved in the second phase of digestion, following chewing. It performs a chemical breakdown due to enzymes and hydrochloric acid.

Stomach

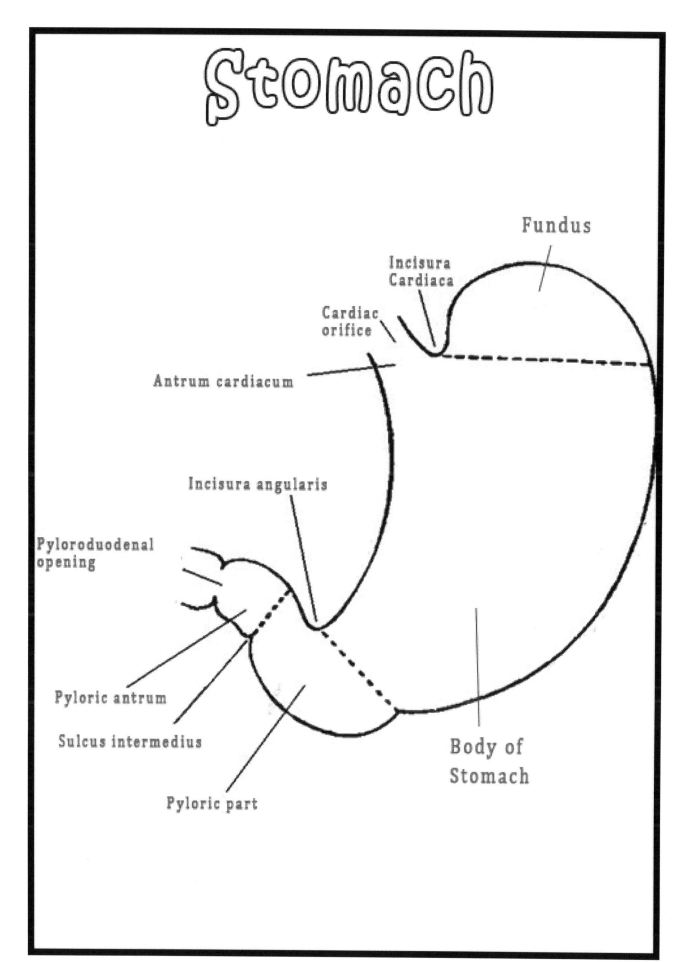

Fundus

Incisura
Cardiaca

Cardiac
orifice

Antrum cardiacum

Incisura angularis

Pyloroduodenal
opening

Pyloric antrum

Sulcus intermedius

Pyloric part

Body of
Stomach

The male reproductive system

consists of a number of sex organs that play a role in the process of human reproduction. These organs are located on the outside of the body and within the pelvis.

The main male sex organs are the penis and the testicles which produce semen and sperm, which, as part of sexual intercourse, fertilize an ovum in the female's body; the fertilized ovum (zygote) develops into a fetus, which is later born as an infant.

Male
Reproductive system

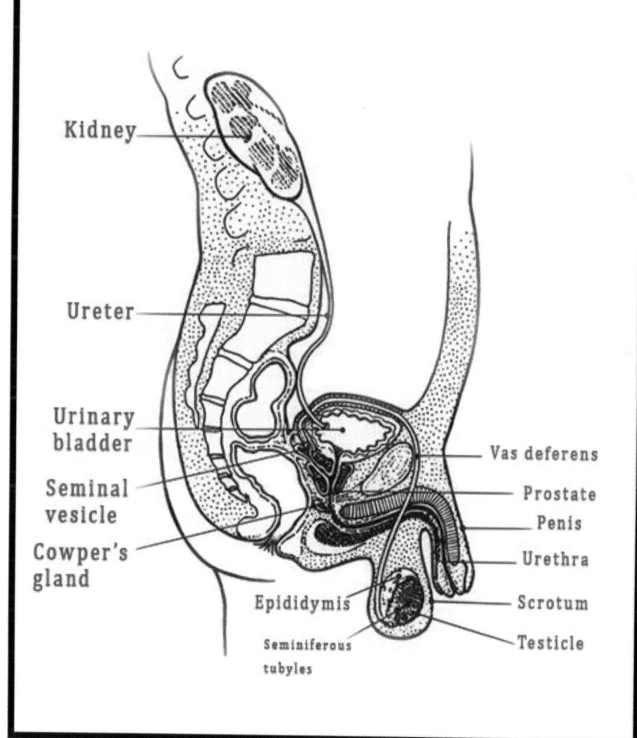

Kidney

Ureter

Urinary
bladder

Seminal
vesicle

Cowper's
gland

Epididymis

Seminiferous
tubyles

Vas deferens

Prostate

Penis

Urethra

Scrotum

Testicle

The **female** reproductive system

consists of a number of sex organs that play a role in the process of human reproduction. These organs are located on the outside of the body and within the pelvis.

Human femal reproductive system:
(Anterior view)

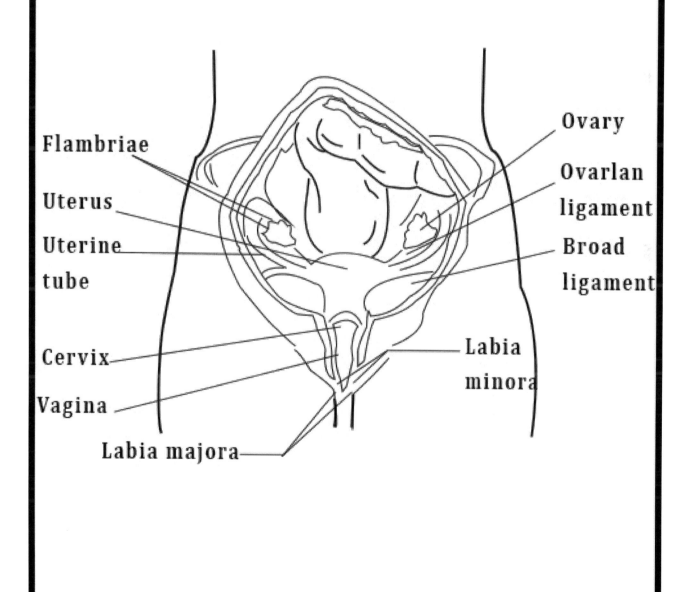

Flambriae

Uterus

Uterine
tube

Cervix

Vagina

Labia majora

Ovary

Ovarlan
ligament

Broad
ligament

Labia
minora

The **female**
reproductive system

The internal sex organs are
the uterus, Fallopian tubes,
and ovaries. The uterus or
womb accommodates the
embryo which develops into
the foetus. The uterus also
produces vaginal and uterine
secretions which help the
transit of sperm to the
Fallopian tubes. The ovaries
produce the ova (egg cells).

Female Reproductive system

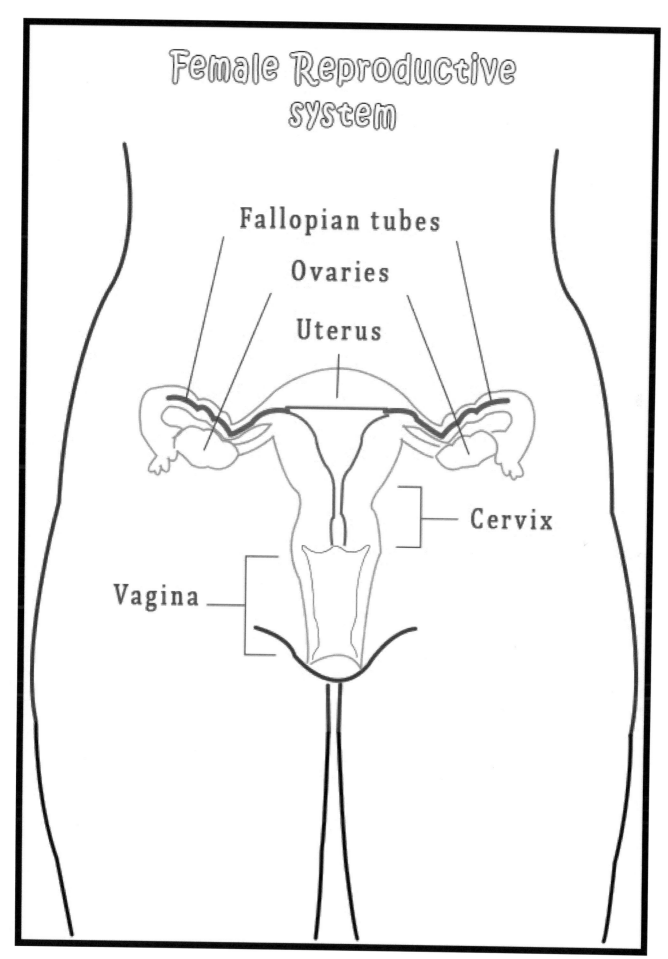

Fallopian tubes

Ovaries

Uterus

Cervix

Vagina

The female reproductive system

The external sex organs are also known as the *genitals* and these are the organs of the vulva including the labia, clitoris, and vaginal opening. The vagina is connected to the uterus at the cervix.

Human femal reproductive system

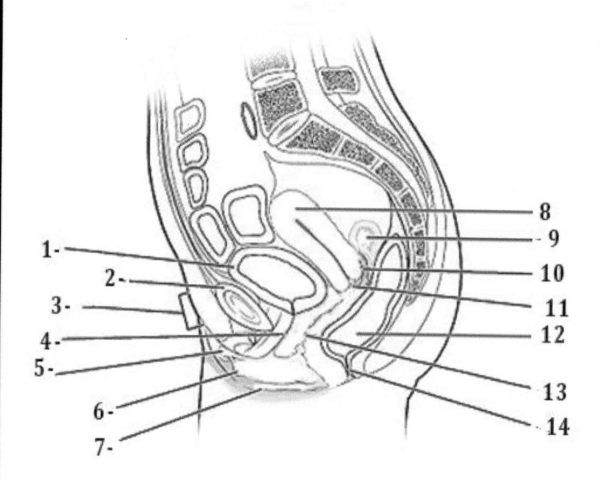

1-
2-
3-
4-
5-
6-
7-

8
9
10
11
12
13
14

1- Bladder

2- Public symphysis

3- Mons pubis

4- Urethra

5- Clitoris

6- Labium minora

7- Labium majora

8- Uteros

9- Ovary

10- Fornix of uterus

11- Cervix

12- Rectum

13- Vagina

14- Anus

The **uterus**

is a major female hormone-responsive secondary sex organ of the reproductive system in humans and most other mammals. In the human, the lower end of the uterus, the cervix, opens into the vagina, while the upper end, the fundus, is connected to the fallopian tubes.

Uterus

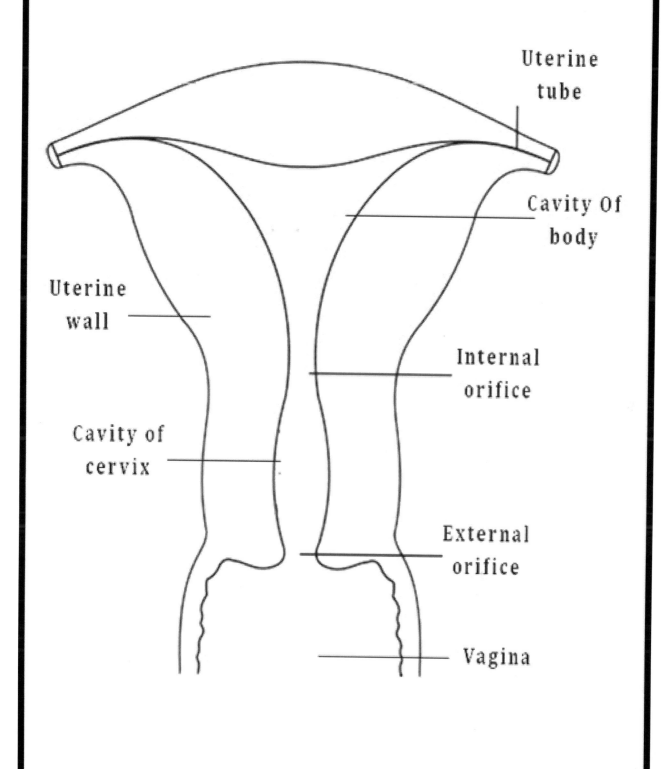

Uterine
tube

Cavity Of
body

Uterine
wall

Internal
orifice

Cavity of
cervix

External
orifice

Vagina

The **breast**

The breast is one of two prominences located on the upper ventral region of the torso of primates. In females, it serves as the mammary gland, which produces and secretes milk to feed infants.

Breast

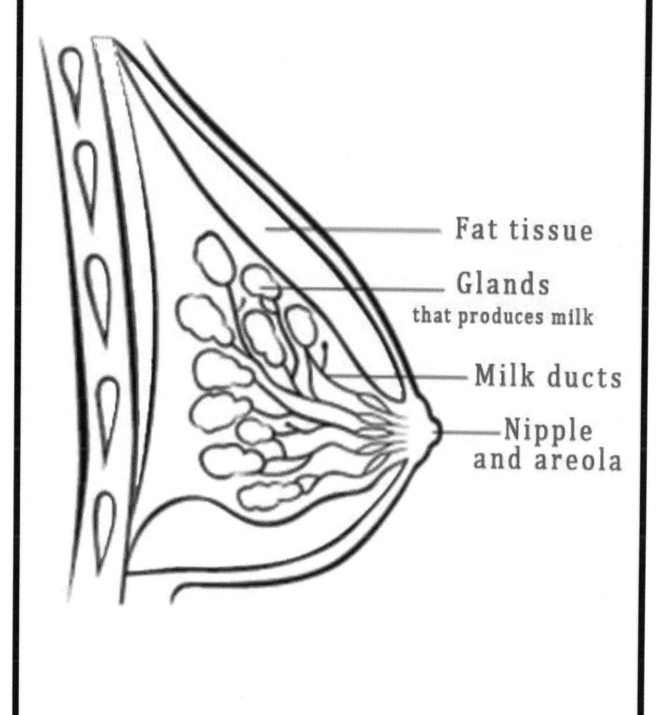

Fat tissue

Glands
that produces milk

Milk ducts

Nipple
and areola

The **pregnancy**

is the time during which one or more offspring develops inside a woman. A multiple pregnancy involves more than one offspring, such as with twins. Pregnancy can occur by sexual intercourse or assisted reproductive technology. A pregnancy may end in a live birth, miscarriage, or abortion.

Pregnancy

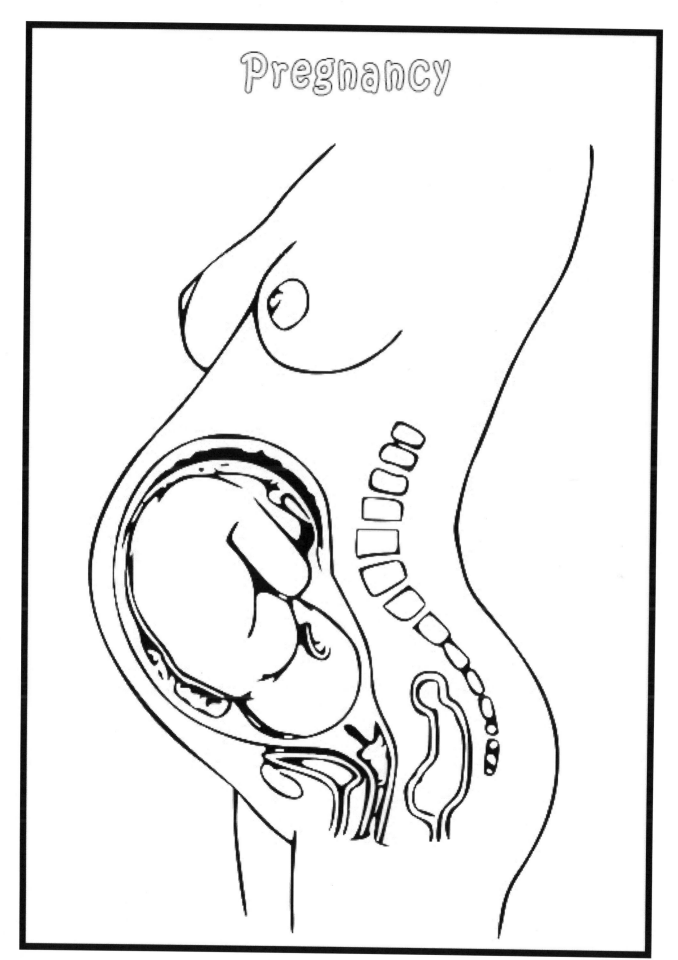

The **five senses**

The five human senses are
the sense of sight, hearing,
touch, smell, and taste.
These five human senses
play a unique role by
receiving signal
information from the
environment through the
sense organs and relaying it
to the human brain for
interpretation.

The five senses

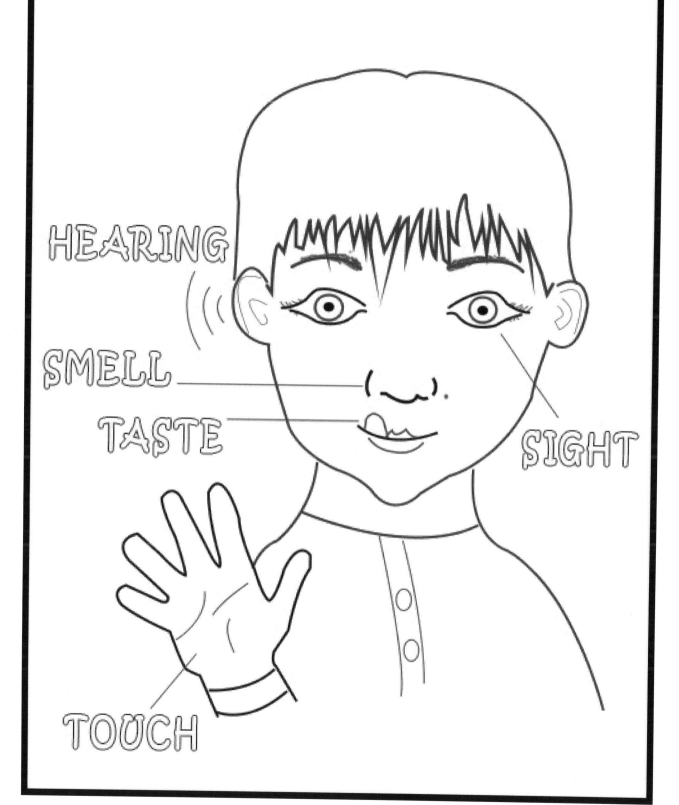

HEARING

SMELL

TASTE

SIGHT

TOUCH

The five senses

are contained in
specially adapted
body sense organs
that include the
eyes, ears, skin, nose,
and the tongue.

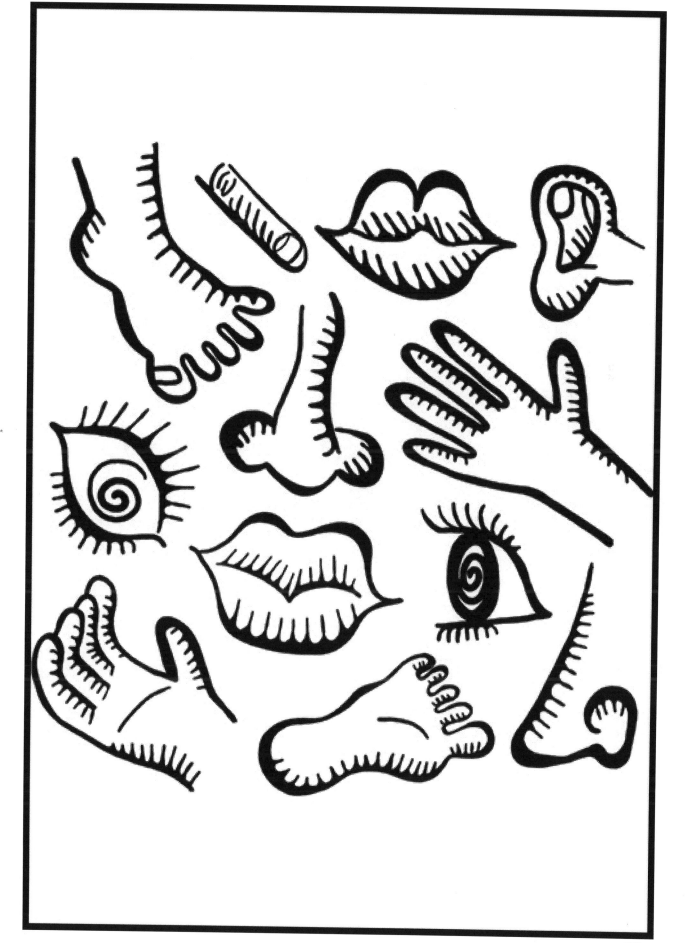

The hand

is a prehensile, multi-fingered appendage located at the end of the forearm or forelimb of primates such as humans, chimpanzees, monkeys, and lemurs.

Hand

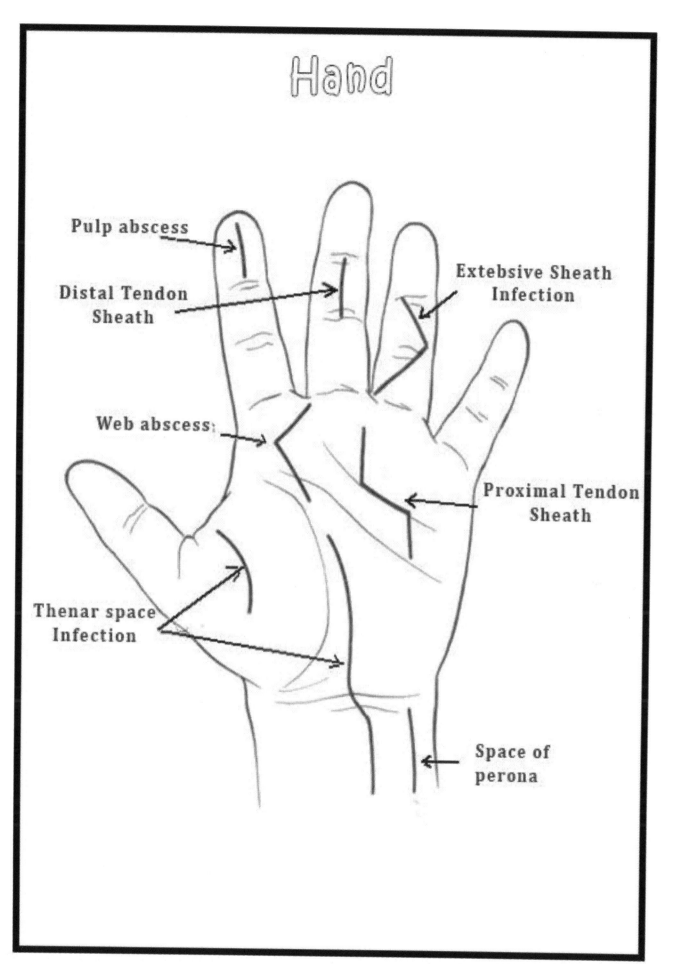

Pulp abscess

Distal Tendon
Sheath

Extebsive Sheath
Infection

Web abscess

Proximal Tendon
Sheath

Thenar space
Infection

Space of
perona

The hand

The skeleton of the human hand consists of 27 bones:

8 Carpals,

5 Metacarpals,

5 Proximal phalanges,

4 Intermediate phalanges,

5 Distal phalanges.

Hand's Joints and Bones

Joints

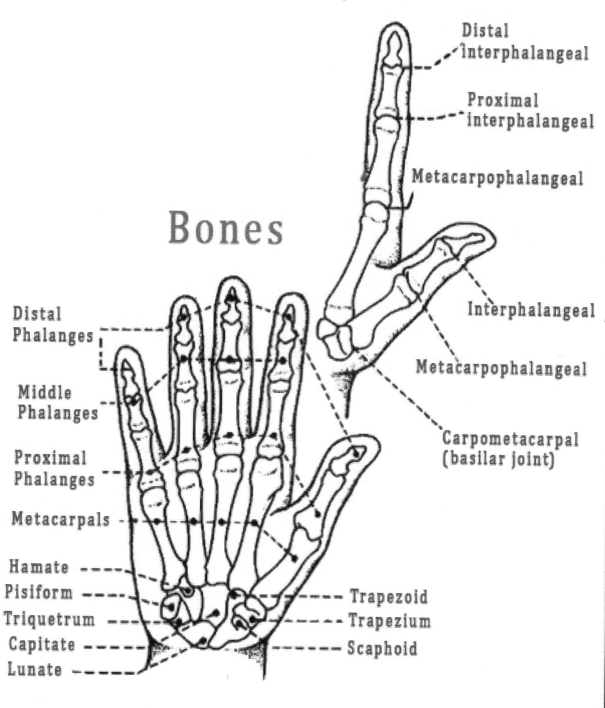

Distal interphalangeal

Proximal interphalangeal

Metacarpophalangeal

Bones

Interphalangeal

Metacarpophalangeal

Carpometacarpal (basilar joint)

Distal Phalanges

Middle Phalanges

Proximal Phalanges

Metacarpals

Hamate

Pisiform

Triquetrum

Capitate

Lunate

Trapezoid

Trapezium

Scaphoid

The **hand gestures**

are a form of nonverbal
communication in which
visible handly actions are
used to communicate
important messages,
either in place of speech
or together and in
parallel with spoken
words.

Hand Gestures

The hand gestures

Some examples:
- *Merkel-Raute.* Described as "probably one of the most recognizable hand gestures in the world", the signature gesture of Angela Merkel has become a political symbol used by both her supporters and opponents.
- Hand heart is a recent pop culture symbol meaning love. The hands form the shape of a heart.
- Thumbs Up and Thumbs Down are common gestures of approval or disapproval made by extending the thumb upward or downward.

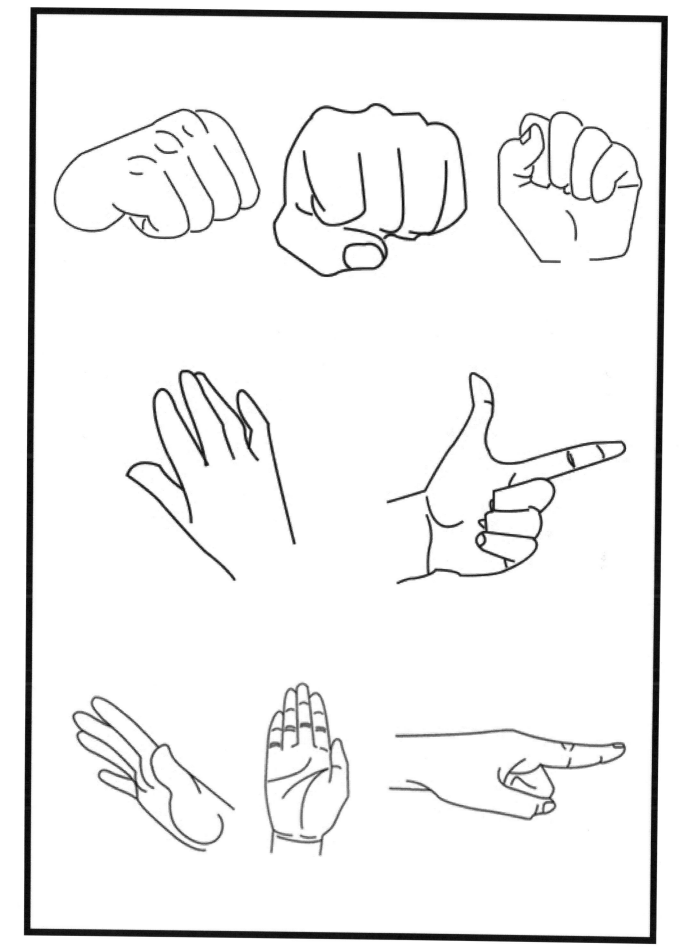

The shoulder

is made up of three bones: the clavicle (collarbone), the scapula (shoulder blade), and the humerus (upper arm bone) as well as associated muscles, ligaments and tendons.

The arm

is the part of the upper limb between the glenohumeral joint (shoulder joint) and the elbow joint.

Shoulder, Arm and Hand

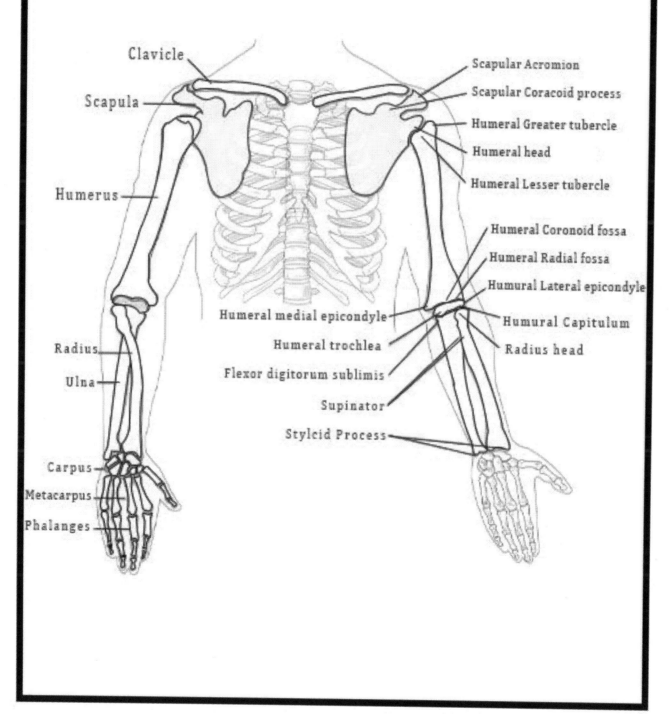

Clavicle

Scapula

Humerus

Radius

Ulna

Carpus

Metacarpus

Phalanges

Scapular Acromion

Scapular Coracoid process

Humeral Greater tubercle

Humeral head

Humeral Lesser tubercle

Humeral Coronoid fossa

Humeral Radial fossa

Humural Lateral epicondyle

Humural Capitulum

Radius head

Humeral medial epicondyle

Humeral trochlea

Flexor digitorum sublimis

Supinator

Stylcid Process

The foot

is an anatomical structure
found in humans. It is the
terminal portion of a limb
which bears weight and
allows locomotion. The
foot is a separate organ at
the terminal part of the
leg made up of one or
more segments or bones,
generally including claws
or nails.

Foot

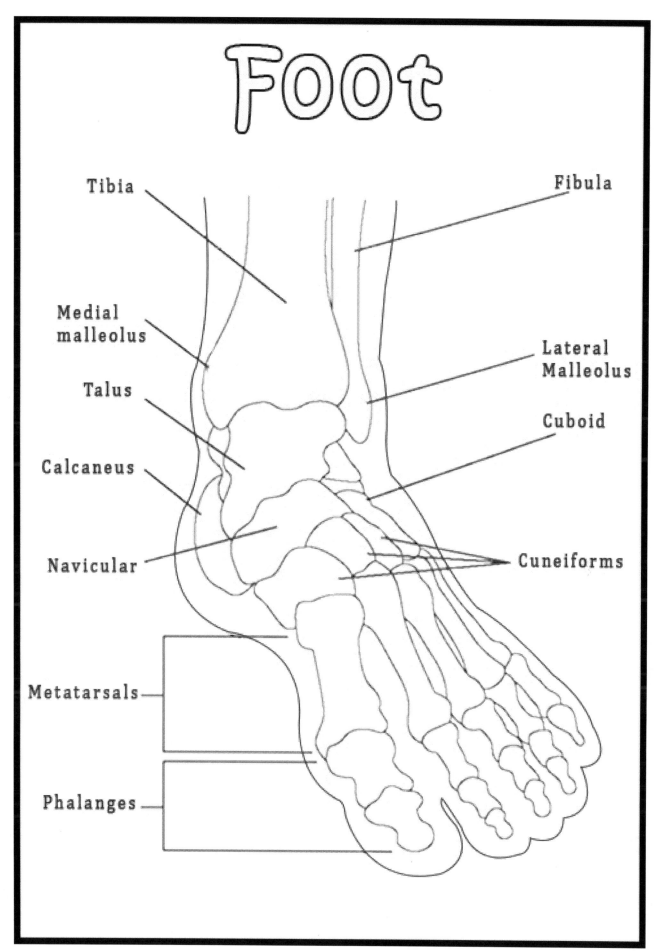

Tibia

Fibula

Medial malleolus

Lateral Malleolus

Talus

Cuboid

Calcaneus

Navicular

Cuneiforms

Metatarsals

Phalanges

The leg

is a weight-bearing and locomotive anatomical structure, usually having a columnar shape. During locomotion, legs function as "extensible struts". The combination of movements at all joints can be modeled as a single, linear element capable of changing length and rotating about an omnidirectional "hip" joint.

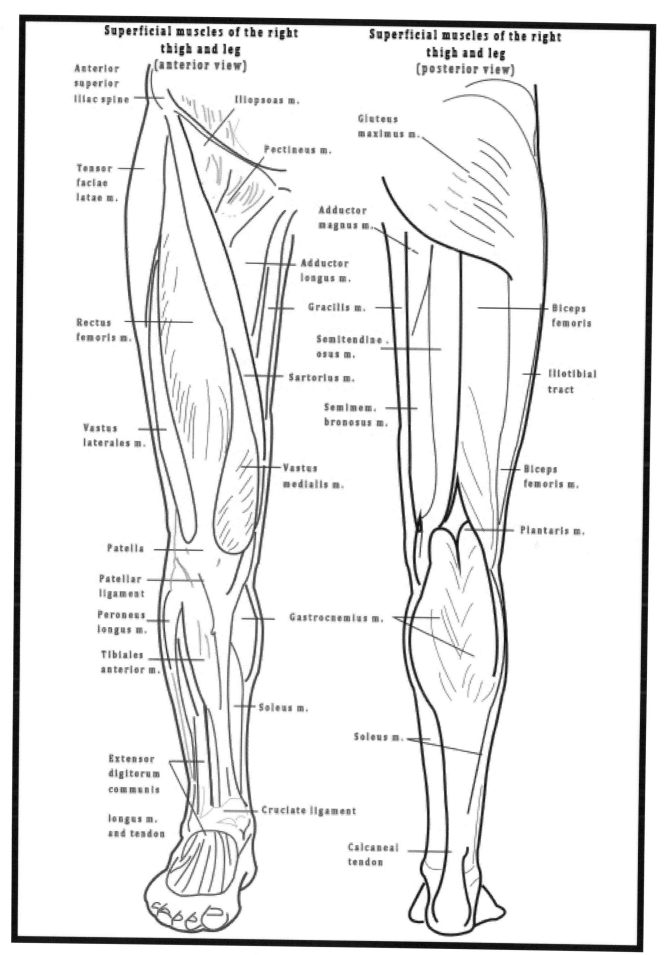

Superficial muscles of the right thigh and leg (anterior view)

Anterior superior iliac spine

Iliopsoas m.

Pectineus m.

Tensor faciae latae m.

Rectus femoris m.

Vastus laterales m.

Vastus medialis m.

Patella

Patellar ligament

Peroneus longus m.

Tibiales anterior m.

Extensor digitorum communis longus m. and tendon

Soleus m.

Cruciate ligament

Adductor longus m.

Gracilis m.

Sartorius m.

Superficial muscles of the right thigh and leg (posterior view)

Gluteus maximus m.

Adductor magnus m.

Semitendine. osus m.

Semimem. bronosus m.

Biceps femoris

Iliotibial tract

Biceps femoris m.

Plantaris m.

Gastrocnemius m.

Soleus m.

Calcaneal tendon

The leg

is a structure of gross anatomy, meaning that it is large enough to be seen unaided. The components depend on the animal. In humans and other mammals, a leg includes the bones, muscles, tendons, ligaments, blood vessels, nerves, and skin. In insects, the leg includes most of these things, except that insects have an exoskeleton that replaces the function of both the bones and the skin.

Superficial pelvic and thigh muscles of right leg (Anterior view)

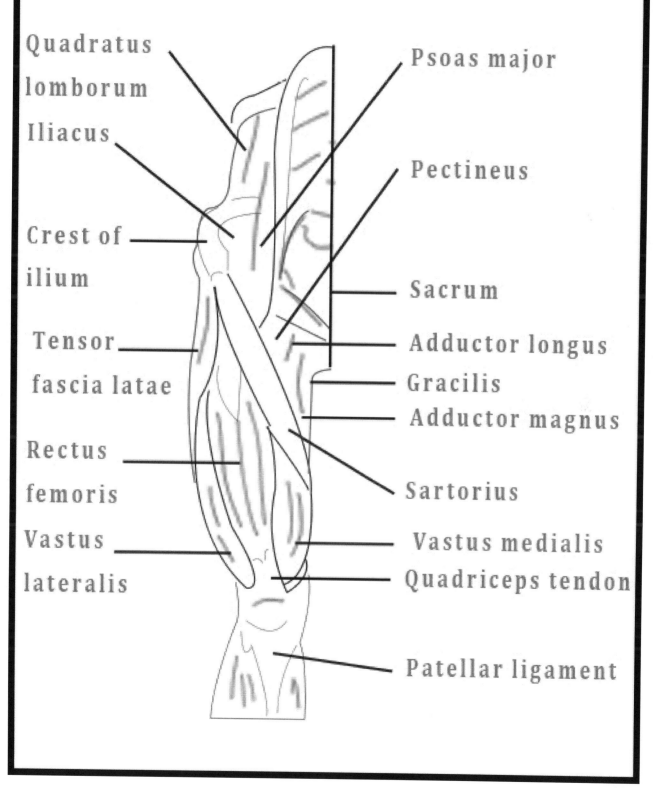

Quadratus lomborum

Iliacus

Crest of ilium

Tensor fascia latae

Rectus femoris

Vastus lateralis

Psoas major

Pectineus

Sacrum

Adductor longus

Gracilis

Adductor magnus

Sartorius

Vastus medialis

Quadriceps tendon

Patellar ligament

The **pelvis**

is either the lower part
of the trunk of the
human body between
the abdomen and the
thighs (sometimes also
called pelvic region of
the trunk) or the
skeleton embedded in it
(sometimes also called
bony pelvis, or pelvic
skeleton).

Pelvic and thigh muscles of right leg
(posterior view)

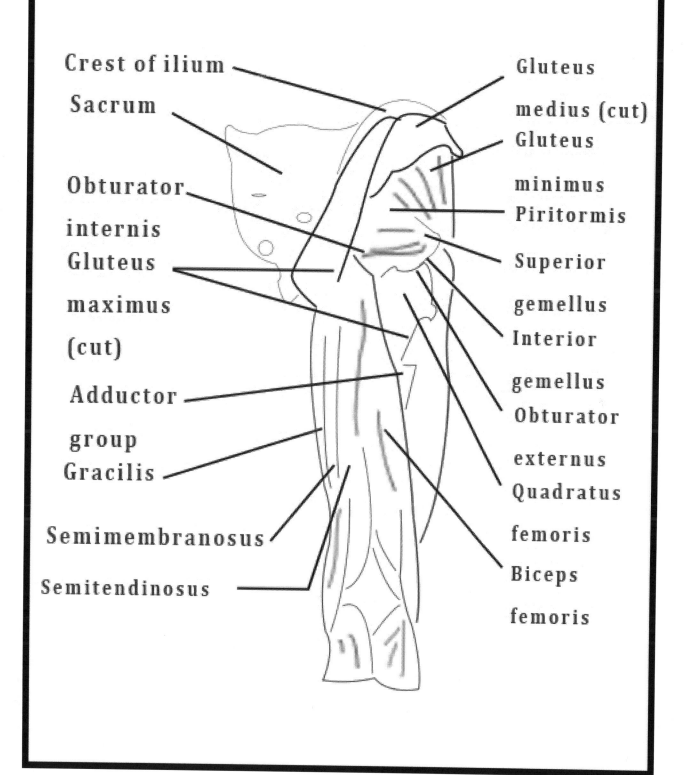

Crest of ilium

Sacrum

Obturator

internis

Gluteus

maximus

(cut)

Adductor

group

Gracilis

Semimembranosus

Semitendinosus

Gluteus

medius (cut)

Gluteus

minimus

Piritormis

Superior

gemellus

Interior

gemellus

Obturator

externus

Quadratus

femoris

Biceps

femoris

The **thigh muscles**

The muscles of the thigh can be classified into three groups according to their location: anterior and posterior muscles and the adductors (on the medial side).

Pelvic and thigh muscles of right leg
(posterior view)

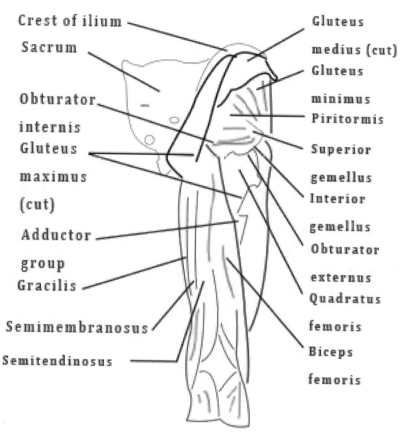

Crest of ilium

Sacrum

Obturator

internis

Gluteus

maximus

(cut)

Adductor

group

Gracilis

Semimembranosus

Semitendinosus

Gluteus

medius (cut)

Gluteus

minimus

Piritormis

Superior

gemellus

Interior

gemellus

Obturator

externus

Quadratus

femoris

Biceps

femoris

Deep pelvic
and thigh muscles
of right leg
(anterior view)

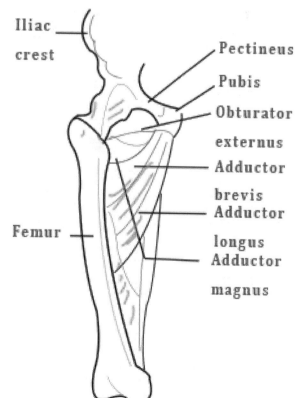

Iliac

crest

Femur

Pectineus

Pubis

Obturator

externus

Adductor

brevis

Adductor

longus

Adductor

magnus

Made in the USA
Middletown, DE
16 October 2023